Delicic

Recipes for

Your Air Fryer

A Healthier Way of Frying.
Cook Your Meals Using Your
Air Fryer to Enjoy Healthier
Food

By

Alice Ramos

This document is geared towards providing exact and reliable information in regards to the topic and issue covered. The publication is sold with the idea that the publisher is not required to render accounting, officially permitted or otherwise qualified services. If advice is necessary, legal or professional, a practiced individual in the profession should be ordered.

From a Declaration of Principles which was accepted and approved equally by a Committee of the American Bar Association and a Committee of Publishers and Associations.

In no way is it legal to reproduce, duplicate, or transmit any part of this document in either electronic means or in printed format. Recording of this publication is strictly prohibited, and any storage of this document is not allowed unless with written permission from the publisher. All rights reserved.

The information provided herein is stated to be truthful and consistent, in that any liability, in terms of inattention or otherwise, by any

contract or any type of guarantee assurance.

The trademarks used are without any consent, and the publication of the trademark is without permission or backing by the trademark owner. All trademarks and brands within this book are for clarifying purposes only and are owned by the owners themselves, not affiliated with this document.

Table of Contents

Introduction 10

.... 14

Chapter 1. Breakfast Recipes 14

1. Breakfast Pea Tortilla 15

2. Raspberry Rolls 17

3. Potato and Leek Frittata 19

4. Espresso Oatmeal 21

5. Mushroom Oatmeal 23

.... 25

Chapter 2. Sides, Snacks, and Appetizers Recipes 25

6. Spinach Balls 26

7. Mushrooms Appetizer 27

8. Cheesy Party Wings 30

9. Cheese Sticks 32

10. Sweet Bacon Snack 34

11. Chicken Rolls 36

12. Tasty Kale and Celery Crackers 38

13. Egg White Chips...40

14. Tuna Cakes..41

15. Calamari and Shrimp Snack 42

....**45**

Chapter 3. Vegetable and Vegetarian Recipes........**45**

16. Masala French Fries 46

17. Dal Mint Kebab................................48

18. Cottage Cheese Croquette.................51

19. Barbeque Corn Sandwich..................54

20. Honey Chili Potatoes 56

21. Burger Cutlet..................................58

22. Pizza 60

23. Cheese French Fries.........................63

....**66**

Chapter 4. Pork, Beef, and Lamb Recipes...............**66**

24. Pudding of Bacon 67

25. Sausage Balls.................................69

26. Cutlets Pork Burger.........................70

27. Venison Garlic................................73

28. Pork Barbecue Sandwich..................74

29. Chili Lamb 77

.... 79

Chapter 5. Fish and Seafood 79

30. Appetizer of Cajun Shrimp 80

31. Crispy Shrimps 81

32. Crab Sticks 82

33. Patties in the Salmon Party 84

34. Shrimp Muffins 86

.... 88

Chapter 6. Poultry Recipes 88

35. Japanese Mixed Chicken 89

36. Succulent Turkey Breast Lunch 91

37. Cream Chicken Stew 93

38. Turkey Cakes 95

39. Coconut and Casserole Chicken 97

40. Turkey Burgers 99

.... 101

Chapter 7. Desserts and Sweets Recipes 101

41. Pajamas Jiggery 102

42. Semolina Pudding 104

43. Date Waffles 105

44. Pudding Times 106

45. Mediterranean Splendor 107

46. Pudding of Guava 109

47. Passion Fruit Pudding 111

48. Blackcurrant Pudding 113

.... 115

Chapter 8. Lunch Recipes 115

49. Whole-Wheat Pizzas in an AirFryer 116

50. Prosciutto Sandwich 118

Conclusion 120

Introduction

One of the most impressive and useful inventions of this decade is undoubtedly the so-called air fryer. It is a machine that arrived on the shelves of the world as the ideal tool to reduce the amount of fat in traditional dishes and snacks such as nuggets and french fries.

Basically, it is an electric appliance that cooks food with hot air, emulating what an ordinary deep fryer would do. It was originally created by the Dutch company Phillips.

Several years after its creation, professional and home cooks seem to have been convinced, and today thousands of brands have replicated the device in different sizes and colors.

The name air fryer may cause confusion in more than one person. Some even wonder which dish is the one with fried air in it. Beyond the bad joke, it seems that the term was given to the device just to make it more attractive and because it appears to replace the conventional frying process.

As such, the verb fry, according to the Royal Spanish Academy, consists of cooking or stewing something in boiling oil or fat, and that is not exactly what the machine does. At most, the maximum amount of oil the air fryer needs is one tablespoon, which is used to coat the food to be cooked, so that it does not stick and forms a crispy crust.

But the machine itself does not fry. It actually cooks with hot air, which makes the food use its own liquids during cooking. The protein or vegetable creates a crispy coating from the contact with the blast of heat, and the inside remains juicy. Therefore, it seems that the final result is a frying, since it maintains the crispiness and color, but, logically, with much less fat.

The utensil has a kind of drawer with a grid in which the food is placed. This can be removed and washed in the dishwasher as normal.

It is not a microwave, since it does not work with electromagnetic waves, nor is it an electric oven, since these do not work with air currents but directly with heat. Therefore, it remains a hot air cooking appliance.

Chapter 1. Breakfast Recipes

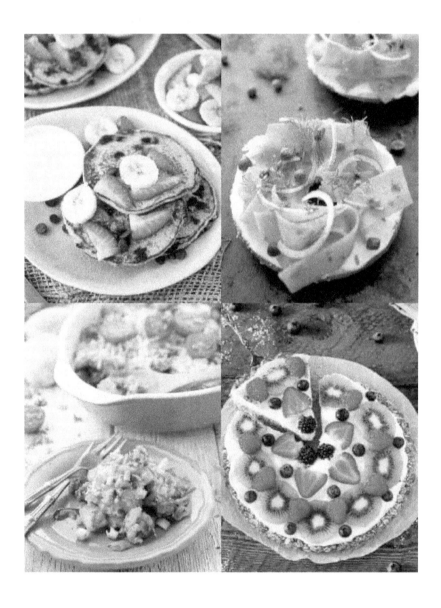

1. Breakfast Pea Tortilla

(Ready in about 17 min | Servings 8 | Easy)

Ingredients:

- ½ pound of baby peas

- 4 tablespoons of butter

- 1 and ½ cup of yogurt

- 8 eggs

- ½ cup of mint, chopped

- Salt and black pepper to the taste

Directions:

1. Heat a saucepan over medium heat that matches your AirFryer with the oil, add peas, stir and cook for a few minutes.

2. Meanwhile, mix half the yogurt with salt, pepper, eggs, and mint in a cup, then whisk well.

3. Pour over the peas, toss, stir in the AirFryer and cook for 7 minutes at 350° F.

4. Pour the remaining yogurt over the tortilla, peel, and serve.

Enjoy!

Nutrition: Calories: 192g, Fat: 5g, Fiber: 4g, Carbs: 8g, Protein: 7g.

2. Raspberry Rolls

(Ready in about 50 min | Servings 6 | Normal)

Ingredients:

- 1 cup of milk

- 4 tablespoons of butter

- 3 and ¼ cups of flour

- 2 teaspoons of yeast

- ¼ cup of sugar

- 1 egg

For the filling:

- 8 ounces of cream cheese, soft

- 12 ounces of raspberries

- 1 teaspoon of vanilla extract

- 5 tablespoons of sugar

- 1 tablespoon of cornstarch

- Zest from 1 lemon, grated

Directions:

1. Mix the flour with the sugar and leaven in a bowl and whisk.

2. Attach milk and egg, stir until a dough is formed, set it aside for 30 minutes to rise, move the dough to a working surface, and roll well.

3. Mix cream cheese with butter, vanilla, and lemon zest in a cup, then stir well and scatter over bread.

4. Mix raspberries and cornstarch in another dish, stir and scatter over it. Combine cream cheese.

5. Shape your bread, break it into small parts, put it in your AirFryer, spray it with a cooking spray, and cook it for 30 minutes at 350° F.

6. Serve for breakfast.

Enjoy!

Nutrition: Calories: 261, Fat: 5g, Fiber: 8g, Carbs: 9g, Protein: 6g.

3. Potato and Leek Frittata

(Ready in about 28 min | Servings 4 | Normal)

Ingredients:

- 2 gold potatoes, boiled, peeled, and chopped

- 2 tablespoons of butter

- 2 leeks, sliced

- Salt and black pepper to the taste

- ¼ cup of whole milk

- 10 eggs, whisked

- 5 ounces of white cheese, crumbled

Directions:

1. Heat a pan over medium heat that suits your AirFryer with the oil, add leeks, stir and cook for 4 minutes.

2. Attach the onions, salt, pepper, bacon, cheese, and butter, whisk well, cook for another 1 minute, put in AirFryer, and cook at 350° F for 13 minutes.

3. Break the frittata into cups, slice, and serve.

Enjoy!

Nutrition: Calories: 271, Fat: 6g, Fiber: 8g, Carbs: 12g, Protein: 6g.

4. Espresso Oatmeal

(Ready in about 27 min | Servings 4 | Normal)

Ingredients:

- 1 cup of milk

- 1 cup of steel-cut oats

- 2 and ½ cups of water

- 2 tablespoons of sugar

- 1 teaspoon of espresso powder

- 2 teaspoons of vanilla extract

Directions:

1. Mix oats with tea, sugar, milk, and espresso powder in a saucepan that suits your AirFryer, stir, place in your AirFryer and cook for 17 minutes at 360° F.

2. Attach the vanilla extract, whisk, set all 5 minutes off, split into bowls and serve.

Enjoy!

Nutrition: Calories: 261, Fat: 7g, Fiber: 6g, Carbs: 39g, Protein: 6g.

5. Mushroom Oatmeal

(Ready in about 30 min | Servings 4 | Normal)

Ingredients:

- 1 small yellow onion, chopped

- 1 cup of steel-cut oats

- 2 garlic cloves, minced

- 2 tablespoons of butter

- ½ cup of water

- 14 ounces of canned chicken stock

- 3 thyme springs, chopped

- 2 tablespoons of extra virgin olive oil

- ½ cup of gouda cheese, grated

- 8 ounces of mushroom, sliced

- Salt and black pepper to the taste

Directions:

1. Heat a pan over medium heat that suits your AirFryer with the butter, add onions and garlic, stir and cook for 4 minutes.

2. Attach oats, sugar, salt, pepper, stock, and thyme, stir, place in the AirFryer and cook for 16 minutes at 360° F.

3. In the meantime, prepare a skillet over medium heat with the olive oil, add mushrooms, cook them for 3 minutes, add oatmeal and cheese, whisk, divide into bowls and serve for breakfast.

Enjoy!

Nutrition: Calories: 284, Fat: 8g, Fiber: 8g, Carbs: 20g, Protein: 17g.

Chapter 2. Sides, Snacks, and Appetizers Recipes

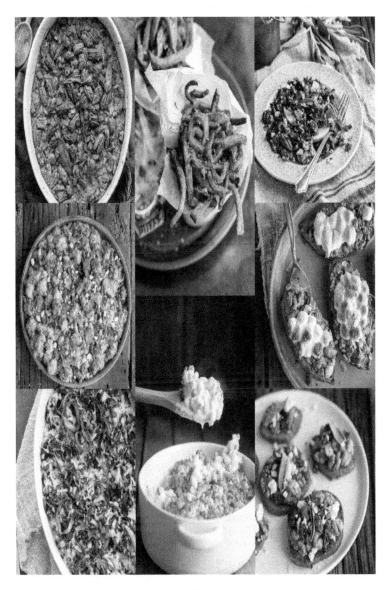

6. Spinach Balls

(Ready in about 17 min | Servings 30 | Normal)

Ingredients:

- 4 tablespoons of butter, melted

- 2 eggs

- 1 cup of flour

- 16 ounces of spinach

- 1/3 cup of feta cheese, crumbled

- ¼ teaspoon of nutmeg, ground

- 1/3 cup of parmesan, grated

- Salt and black pepper to the taste

- 1 tablespoon of onion powder

- 3 tablespoons of whipping cream

- 1 teaspoon of garlic powder

Directions:

1. Mix spinach with butter, milk, pasta, feta cheese, parmesan, nutmeg, whipped cream, salt, pepper, onion, and garlic powder in your blender, mix very well and carry for 10 minutes in the freezer.

2. Shape 30 spinach balls, put them in the basket of your AirFryer, and cook for 7 minutes at 300° F.

3. Serve as an appetizer to a crowd.

Enjoy!

Nutrition: Calories: 60, Fat: 5g, Fiber: 1g, Carbs: 1g, Protein: 2g.

7. Mushrooms Appetizer

(Ready in about 20 min | Servings 4 | Normal)

Ingredients:

- ¼ cup of mayonnaise

- 1 teaspoon of garlic powder

- 1 small yellow onion, chopped

- 24 ounces of white mushroom caps

- Salt and black pepper to the taste

- 1 teaspoon of curry powder

- 4 ounces of cream cheese, soft

- ¼ cup of sour cream

- ½ cup of Mexican cheese, shredded

- 1 cup of shrimp, cooked, peeled, deveined, and chopped

Directions:

1. Mix mayo to blend and shake well in a bowl with garlic powder, onion, curry powder, cream cheese, sour cream, Mexican cheese, seafood, salt, and pepper.

2. Stuff the mushrooms with this mixture put them in the basket from your AirFryer, and cook for 10 minutes at 300° F.

3. Arrange on a tray and serve as an appetizer.

Enjoy!

Nutrition: Calories: 200, Fat: 20g, Fiber: 3g, Carbs: 16g, Protein: 14g.

8. Cheesy Party Wings

(Ready in about 22 min | Servings 6 | Normal)

Ingredients:

- 6-pound of chicken wings, halved

- Salt and black pepper to the taste

- ½ teaspoon of Italian seasoning

- 2 tablespoons of butter

- ½ cup parmesan of cheese, grated

- A pinch of red pepper flakes, crushed

- 1 teaspoon of garlic powder

- 1 egg

Directions:

1. Arrange chicken wings in the tray of your AirFryer and roast for 9 minutes at 390° F.

2. Meanwhile, mix butter with cheese, milk, salt, pepper, pepper flakes, garlic powder, and Italian seasoning in your blender and combine well.

3. Take out chicken wings, pour over the cheese sauce, swirl well to coat, and cook for 3 minutes in your AirFryer's basket at 390° F.

4. Serve like an appetizer to them.

Enjoy!

Nutrition: Calories: 204, Fat: 8g, Fiber: 1g, Carbs: 18g, Protein: 14g.

9. Cheese Sticks

(Ready in about 1hr 18 min | Servings 16 | Normal)

Ingredients:

- 2 eggs, whisked

- Salt and black pepper to the taste

- 8 mozzarella cheese strings, cut into halves

- 1 cup of parmesan, grated

- 1 tablespoon of Italian seasoning

- Cooking spray

- 1 garlic clove, minced

Directions:

1. Grab a package of mozzarella string cheese and cut each of the sticks in half. Place them into a baggie and freeze. Arrange the cheese in

the tray of your AirFryer and roast for 9 minutes at 390° F.

2. Freeze them, so the outside has a chance to get crispy before the cheese melts too much.

3. Air fry! All you do is pre-heat, place the mozzarella stick into the AirFryer, and "fry" for 5 minutes.

4. Serve like as an appetizer.

Enjoy!

Nutrition: Calories: 140, Fat: 5g, Fiber: 1g, Carbs: 3g, Protein: 4g.

10. Sweet Bacon Snack

(Ready in about 40 min | Servings 16 | Normal)

Ingredients:

- ½ teaspoon of cinnamon powder

- 16 bacon slices

- 1 tablespoon of avocado oil

- 3 ounces of dark chocolate

- 1 teaspoon of maple extract

Directions:

1. Arrange bacon slices in the AirFryer basket, sprinkle the cinnamon mixture over them, and prepare them for 30 minutes at 300° F.

2. Heat a pot over medium heat with the oil, add the chocolate and stir until it melts.

3. Add extract of the syrup, mix, take off the heat, and allow to cool down a little.

4. Take the bacon strips out of the oven, leave them to cool down, dip each in a mixture of chocolate, put them on parchment paper, and let them cool down.

5. Serve as a snack, like ice.

Enjoy!

Nutrition: Calories: 200, Fat: 4g, Fiber: 5g, Carbs: 12g, Protein: 3g.

11. Chicken Rolls

(Ready in about 2hr 20 min | Servings 16 | Normal)

Ingredients:

- 4 ounces of blue cheese, crumbled

- 2 cups of chicken, cooked and chopped

- Salt and black pepper to the taste

- 2 green onions, chopped

- 2 celery stalks, finely chopped

- ½ cup of tomato sauce

- 12 egg roll wrappers

- Cooking spray

Directions:

1. Mix chicken meat with blue cheese, salt, pepper, green onions, celery, and tomato sauce in

a cup, then mix well and hold for 2 hours in the refrigerator.

2. Drop egg wrappers onto a working board, cut the chicken blend, roll and seal edges on them.

3. Put rolls in the basket of your AirFryer, spray them with the cooking oil, and cook them for 10 minutes at 350° F, flipping them halfway.

Enjoy!

Nutrition: Calories: 220, Fat: 7g, Fiber: 2g, Carbs: 14g, Protein: 10g.

12. Tasty Kale and Celery Crackers

(Ready in about 30 min | Servings 6 | Normal)

Ingredients:

- 2 cups of flaxseed, ground

- 2 cups of flax seed, soaked overnight and drained

- 4 bunches of kale, chopped

- 1 bunch of basil, chopped

- ½ bunch of celery, chopped

- 4 garlic cloves, minced

- 1/3 cup of olive oil

Directions:

1. Mix the ground flaxseed with the celery, kale, basil, and garlic in your food processor and mix well.

2. Add the oil and soaked flaxseed, then mix again, scatter in the pan of your AirFryer, break into medium crackers and cook for 20 minutes at 380° F.

3. Serve as an appetizer and break into cups.

Enjoy!

Nutrition: Calories: 143, Fat: 1g, Fiber: 2g, Carbs: 8g, Protein: 4g.

13. Egg White Chips

(Ready in about 13 min | Servings 2 | Normal)

Ingredients:

- ½ tablespoon of water

- 2 tablespoons of parmesan, shredded

- 4 eggs whites

- Salt and black pepper to the taste

Directions:

1. Mix the egg whites with salt, pepper, and water in a cup, then whisk well.

2. Sprinkle this in a muffin tin that suits your AirFryer, sprinkle the cheese on top, fill in the AirFryer and cook for 8 minutes at 350° F.

3. Arrange white egg chips on a plate and serve as a snack.

Enjoy!

Nutrition: Calories: 180, Fat: 2g, Fiber: 1g, Carbs: 12g, Protein: 7g.

14. Tuna Cakes

(Ready in about 20 min | Servings 12 | Normal)

Ingredients:

- 15 ounces of canned tuna, drain and flaked

- 3 eggs

- ½ teaspoon of dill, dried

- 1 teaspoon of parsley, dried

- ½ cup of red onion, chopped

- 1 teaspoon of garlic powder

- Salt and black pepper to the taste

- Cooking spray

Directions:

1. Mix the tuna with salt, pepper, dill, parsley, onion, garlic powder, and eggs in a cup, whisk well, and make medium cakes out of the mixture.

2. Place the tuna cakes in the basket of your AirFryer, spray them with the cooking oil and cook for 10 minutes at 350° F and turn them halfway.

3. Place them on a tray and act as an appetizer.

Enjoy!

15. Calamari and Shrimp Snack

(Ready in about 30 min | Servings 1 | Normal)

Ingredients:

- 8 ounces of calamari, cut into medium rings

- 7 ounces of shrimp, peeled and deveined

- 1 egg

- 3 tablespoons of white flour

- 1 tablespoon of olive oil

- 2 tablespoons of avocado, chopped

- 1 teaspoon of tomato paste

- 1 tablespoon of mayonnaise

- A splash of Worcestershire sauce

- 1 teaspoon of lemon juice

- Salt and black pepper to the taste

- ½ teaspoon of turmeric powder

Directions:

1. Whisk the egg with oil in a mug, apply the calamari and shrimp rings, and toss to cover.

2. Mix the flour with salt, pepper, and turmeric in another dish, then whisk.

3. In this combination, dredge calamari and shrimp, put them in the basket of your AirFryer,

and cook for 9 minutes at 350° F, flipping them once.

4. Meanwhile, blend avocado with tomato paste and mayo in a cup, and mash with a fork.

5. Stir well and apply Worcestershire sauce, lemon juice, salt, and pepper.

6. Arrange calamari and shrimp on a tray, then serve horizontally with the sauce.

Enjoy!

Nutrition: Calories: 288, Fat: 23g, Fiber: 3g, Carbs: 10g, Protein: 15g.

Chapter 3. Vegetable and Vegetarian Recipes

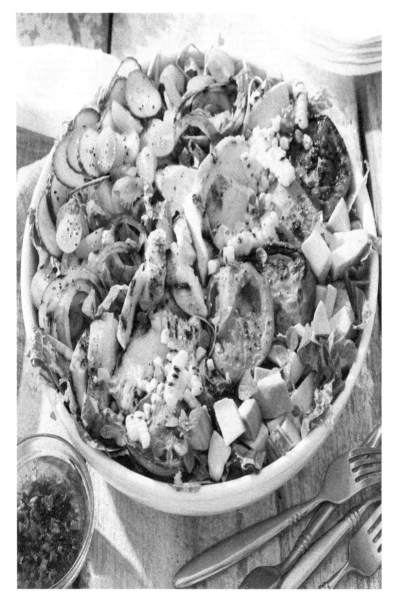

16. Masala French Fries

(Ready in about 30 min | Servings 1 | Normal)

Ingredients:

- 2 medium-sized potatoes peeled and cut into thick pieces lengthwise

Ingredients for the marinade:

- 1 tbsp. of olive oil

- 1 tsp. of mixed herbs

- ½ tsp. of red chili flakes

- A pinch of salt to taste

- 1 tbsp. of lemon juice

Directions:

1. Boil, and blanch the potatoes — split fingertips through the potato. Mix the marinade ingredients

and apply the potato fingers to it, meaning they are well cooked.

2. At 300 Fahrenheit, Preheat the AirFryer for around 5 minutes. Take out the fryer bowl and put the potato fingers in it. Lock the box. Still, hold the fryer for 20 to 25 minutes at 200 Fahrenheit.

3. Toss the fries twice or thrice during the process so they'll be cooked properly.

Nutrition: Calories: 265 kcal.

17. Dal Mint Kebab

(Ready in about 35 min | Servings 2 | Normal)

Ingredients:

- 1 cup of chickpeas

- Half inch ginger grated or one and a half tsp. of ginger-garlic paste

- 1-2 green chilies chopped finely

- ¼ tsp. of red chili powder

- A pinch of salt to the taste

- ½ tsp. of roasted cumin powder

- 2 tsp. of coriander powder

- 1 ½ tbsp. of chopped coriander

- ½ tsp. of dried mango powder

- 1 cup of dry breadcrumbs

- ¼ tsp. of black pepper

- 1-2 tbsp. of all-purpose flour for coating purposes

- 1-2 tbsp. of mint (finely chopped)

- 1 onion that has been finely chopped

- ½ cup of milk

Directions:

1. Take a free vessel. Boil the chickpeas inside the vessel until they become smooth in texture. Made sure they don't get soggy. Now take the chickpea in a separate tub.

2. Apply the ginger rubbed, and the chilies sliced orange. Grind the mixture until it turns into a smooth paste. Continue adding water as and when appropriate. Now add the onions, the mint, the breadcrumbs, and all the different masalas required.

3. Mix until the dough is smooth. Now make small balls from this mix (about the size of a lemon) and form them into flat and circular kebab shape. This is where milk comes in. To soak it, spill a very small amount of milk onto each kebab. Now fold the kebab into the crumbs of dry bread.

4. About 300 Fahrenheit, Preheat the AirFryer for 5 minutes. Take out your bowl. Arrange kebabs in the basket such that no two kebabs hit each other, leaving holes between them. Hold the fryer for about half an hour, at 340 Fahrenheit.

5. Turn the kebabs over halfway through the cooking process so that they can be cooked properly. Mint chutney, tomato ketchup, or yogurt chutney are preferred sides for this sauce.

Nutrition: Calories: 150 kcal.

18. Cottage Cheese Croquette

(Ready in about 25 min | Servings 2 | Normal)

Ingredients:

- 2 cups cottage cheese cut into slightly thick and long pieces (similar to french fries)

- 1 big capsicum (Cut this capsicum into big cubes)

- 1 onion (Cut it into quarters. Now separate the layers carefully.)

- 5 tbsp. of gram flour

- A pinch of salt to the taste

For chutney:

- 2 cups of fresh green coriander

- ½ cup of mint leaves

- 4 tsp. of fennel

- 1 small onion

- 2 tbsp. of ginger-garlic paste

- 6-7 garlic flakes (optional)

- 3 tbsp. of lemon juice

- Salt

Directions:

1. Take a tub that is clean and dry. Put the cilantro, basil, fennel and ginger, onion/garlic, salt, and lemon juice into it. Match and combine.

2. Load the mixture into a grinder, then blend until a smooth paste is produced. So move on to slices of cottage cheese. Cut these bits nearly to the edge, and set them aside. Now stuff all the bits with the paste which was there obtained from the preceding stage. Now set the cottage cheese packed aside.

3. Take the chutney and add some salt and gram flour to it. Mix the two. Rub this blend all over the

stuffed bits of cottage cheese. Now set out the cottage cheese. Now apply the capsicum and onions to the remaining chutney. Gently spread the chutney on each of the capsicum and onion bits. Now take satay sticks and put on different sticks, the cottage cheese bits, and vegetables.

4. At 290 Fahrenheit, Preheat the AirFryer for around 5 minutes. Arrange well the satay holds. Lock the box. Hold the sticks at 180° with the cottage cheese for about half an hour while the sticks with the vegetables are only to be held at the same temperature for 7 minutes.

5. Switch the sticks in between so that one side doesn't get burnt, and a standard cook is also given.

Nutrition: Calories: 160 kcal.

19. Barbeque Corn Sandwich

(Ready in about 40 min | Servings 2 | Normal)

Ingredients:

- 2 slices of white bread

- 1 tbsp. of softened butter

- 1 cup of sweet corn kernels

- 1 small capsicum

For Barbeque Sauce:

- ¼ tbsp. of Worcestershire sauce

- ½ tsp. of olive oil

- ½ flake garlic crushed

- ¼ cup of chopped onion

- ¼ tbsp. of red chili sauce

- ½ cup of water

Directions:

1. Take the bread slices and cut the rims. Still cut horizontally on the strips. Heat the sauce ingredients and wait before the sauce thickens. Now apply the corn to the sauce and stir before the flavors are obtained.

2. Whisk the capsicum and scrape off the flesh. The capsicum is sliced into strips. Apply the sauce to the trimmings. Preheat the AirFryer to 300 Fahrenheit for 5 minutes.

3. Open the Fryer's basket and put the cooked sandwiches in it, ensuring that no two sandwiches meet each other. Hold the fryer at about 15 minutes now at 250°.

4. Switch the sandwiches in-between method of cooking heat slices of both. Serve the strawberry ketchup or mint chutney sandwiches.

Nutrition: Calories: 130 kcal.

20. Honey Chili Potatoes

(Ready in about 25 min | Servings 2 | Normal)

Ingredients:

For potato:

- 3 big potatoes (Cut into strips or cubes)

- 2 ½ tsp. of ginger-garlic paste

- ¼ tsp. of salt

- 1 tsp. of red chili sauce

- ¼ tsp. of red chili powder/black pepper

- A few drops of edible orange food coloring

For sauce:

- 1 capsicum, cut into thin and long pieces (lengthwise).

- 2 tbsp. of olive oil

- 2 onions. Cut them into halves.

- 1 ½ tbsp. of sweet chili sauce

- 1 ½ tsp. of ginger garlic paste

- ½ tbsp. of red chili sauce.

- 2 tbsp. of tomato ketchup

- 2 tsp. of soy sauce

- 2 tsp. of vinegar

- A pinch of black pepper powder

- 1-2 tsp. of red chili flakes

Directions:

1. Creating the potato finger mix and well brushing the chicken with it. Preheat the AirFryer for 5 minutes or so, at 250 Fahrenheit. Attach the Fryer's Box.

2. Place your cubes inside the bowl. Now let the fryer have another 20 minutes to sit at 290 Fahrenheit. Keep flipping your fingers around the cook regularly to get an even fry.

3. Apply the spices to the sauce and apply the vegetables until it thickens. Attach the fingers to the sauce, and simmer until the tastes combine.

Nutrition: Calories: 255 kcal.

21. Burger Cutlet

(Ready in about 25 min | Servings 2 | Normal)

Ingredients:

- 1 large potato boiled and mashed

- ½ cup of breadcrumbs

- A pinch of salt to the taste

- ¼ tsp. of ginger finely chopped

- 1 green chili finely chopped

- 1 tsp. of lemon juice

- 1 tbsp. of fresh coriander leaves. Chop them finely

- ¼ tsp. of red chili powder

- ½ cup of boiled peas

- ¼ tsp. of cumin powder

- ¼ tsp. of dried mango powder

Directions:

1. Mix with the ingredients to make sure the colors are correct. Now you're going to make round cutlets with the mixture and well stretch them out.

2. Preheat the AirFryer for 5 minutes, at 250 Fahrenheit. Open the Fryer basket and place the cutlets within the bowl.

3. Hold the fryer at about 10 to 12 minutes, at 150°. Turn the cutlets over to get a uniform cook in between the cooking process. Serve sweet chutney with basil.

Nutrition: Calories: 177 kcal.

22. Pizza

(Ready in about 40 min | Servings 3 | Easy)

Ingredients:

- One pizza base

- Grated pizza cheese (mozzarella cheese preferably) for topping

- Use cooking oil for brushing and topping purposes

Ingredients for topping:

- 2 onions chopped

- 2 capsicums chopped

- 2 tomatoes that have been deseeded and chopped

- 1 tbsp. (optional) of mushrooms/corns

- 2 tsp. of pizza seasoning

- Some cottage cheese that has been cut into small cubes (optional)

Directions:

1. Place the pizza base for around 5 minutes in a pre-heated AirFryer. (Heated pre to 340 Fahrenheit). Let a foundation back. Place some pizza sauce in the middle on the rim.

2. Pour the sauce around the base using a spoon to make sure you have a distance across the circumference. Grate some mozzarella cheese and scatter on a base of the sauce.

3. Take all the vegetables mentioned above and combine them in a dish. Apply some oil and season to taste. Add a little salt and pepper to taste too. Fit them as well. Place this topping on the pizza over the cheese plate. Now brush over this layer with some more grated cheese and pizza seasoning.

4. Preheat the AirFryer for about 5 minutes, at 250 Fahrenheit. Open the basket with fry and put the

pizza inside. Cover the basket and hold the fryer for another 10 minutes, at 170°. If you thought it is undercooked, you can schedule it for another 2 minutes or so simultaneously.

Nutrition: Calories: 267 kcal.

23. Cheese French Fries

(Ready in about 35 min | Servings 4 | Normal)

Ingredients:

- 2 medium-sized potatoes peeled and cut into thick pieces lengthwise

Ingredients for the marinade:

- 1 tbsp. of olive oil

- 1 tsp. of mixed herbs

- ½ tsp. of red chili flakes

- A pinch of salt to the taste

- 1 tbsp. of lemon juice

For the garnish:

- 1 cup of melted cheddar cheese (You could put this into a piping bag and create a fries pattern.)

Directions:

1. Take all of the listed ingredients under the heading "For the Marinade" and blend well.

2. Now dump 3 cups of water into a tub. In the water, apply a touch of salt. Bring it to the boil. Now blanch the potato bits for about 5 minutes — drain water through a sieve.

3. Dry the bits of potato into a plate and placed them on another dry towel. Cover with the marinade made in the previous phase these potato fingers with.

4. At 300 Fahrenheit, preheat the AirFryer for around 5 minutes. Take out the fryer bowl and put the potato fingers in it. Lock the box.

5. Currently hold the fryer for 20 to 25 minutes at 220 Fahrenheit. Toss the fries twice or thrice during the process so they'll be cooked properly. Sprinkle the cut coriander leaves on the fries at the cooking process (the last 2 minutes or so). Place the cheddar cheese spread over the fries, and serve sweet.

Nutrition: Calories: 335 kcal.

Chapter 4. Pork, Beef, and Lamb Recipes

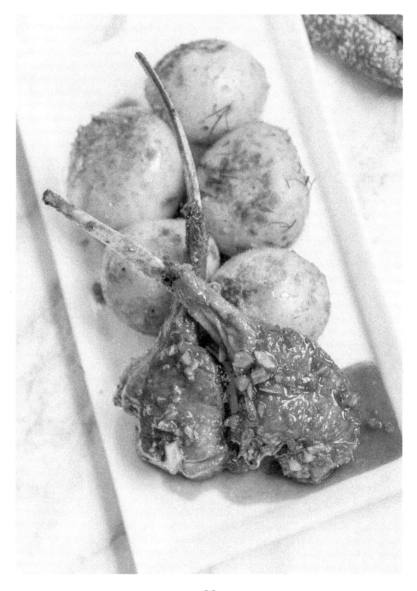

24. Pudding of Bacon

(Ready in about 40 min | Servings 6 | Normal)

Ingredients:

- Four slices of bacon, fried and chopped

- 1 ginger butter, mild

- 2 cups of maize

- One yellow onion, sliced

- Celery: 1/4 cup, chopped

- 1/2 cup of red pepper, sliced

- 1 teaspoon of thyme, cut

- 2 teaspoons of garlic, diced

- Salt and black chili, to try

- 1/2 cup of milk, hard

- 1 and a half cups of milk

- Three whisked eggs

- 3 cups of bread, wrapped

- Four parmesan spoons, rubberized coating

- Cooking spray

Directions:

1. Lubricate the pan with cooking spray on your AirFryer.

2. Comb the bacon in a bowl of butter, corn, onion, pepper bell, celery, thyme, garlic, salt, hot pepper, milk, cream, eggs, and bread. Toss the balls, pour in the grated saucepan, and scatter over the cheese

3. Transfer this to the hot oven 320° AirFryer and cook for 30 minutes

4. Divide between dishes, and serve hot for an easy lunch.

Enjoy!

Nutrition: Calories: 276, Fat: 10g, Carbohydrates 20g, Protein: 10g.

25. Sausage Balls

(Preparation time: 10 min | Cooking time 10 min | Servings 6)

Ingredients:

- 4 ounces of sausage meat, ground

- Salt and black chili, to try

- 1 teaspoon of sage

- 1/2 teaspoon of ginger

- 1 thin, chopped onion

- Three tablespoons of sliced bread

Directions:

1. In a cup, add salt, pepper, ginger, garlic, onion, and cabbage. Mix well breadcrumbs, and make little balls out of this mix.

2. Place them in the basket of your AirFryer and cook at 360° F for 15 minutes. Divide into bowls, then serve as a snack.

Enjoy!

Nutrition: Calories: 130, Fat: 7g, Fiber: 1g, Carbohydrates 13g, Protein: 4g.

26. Cutlets Pork Burger

(Ready in about 30 min | Servings 7 | Normal)

Ingredients:

- 1/2 pounds of pork (Make sure the pork is thinning fine)

- 1/2 cup of diced bread

- A sprinkle of salt

- 1/4 tsp of small chopped ginger

- 1 thinly sliced green chili

- 1 tsp of lemon extract

- 1 tbsp of coriander leaves chop them thinly

- 1/4 tsp powdered red chili

- 1/2 cup of cooked peas

- 1/4 tsp of ground cumin

- 1/4 tsp of dried powdered mango

Directions:

1. Take a container and spill all the masalas, onions, green chilies, peas into it, cilantro leaves, lemon juice, 1-2 tbsp of ginger, and breadcrumbs. Add minced pork. Combine all the ingredients.

2. Mold the combination into Cutlets Round. Press them swiftly. Then roll them out.

3. Preheat the AirFryer for five minutes, at 250 Fahrenheit. Open the basket of the Fryer, then place the Cutlets in the bowl.

4. Hold on the fryer for about 10 to 12 minutes, at 150°. Between the cooking phase, turn over the

Cutlets and get a standardized cook. Serve warm with mint chutney.

Nutrition: Calories: 99, Fat: 10g, Carbohydrates 20g, Protein: 10g.

27. Venison Garlic

(Ready in about 12hr 25 min | Servings 6 | Difficult)

Ingredients:

- 1 lb of boneless venison sliced into fingers

- 2 cups of dried breadcrumbs

- 2 tsp of oregano

- 2 tsp of red pepper flakes

- 2 tsp of garlic Paste

Marinade:

- 1 1/2 tbsp of ginger-garlic paste

- Four tbsp of lemon extract

- 2 tsp of salt

- 1 tsp of powdered red chili

- Six tbsp of cornflour

- 4 eggs

Directions:

1. Combine all of the marinade ingredients and bring the venison fingers inside and let it rest overnight.

2. Comb well the flakes of breadcrumbs, oregano, and red chili, and put the fingers brined on this paste. Cover with plastic wrap and leave before serve to cook.

3. Pre fire up the AirFryer for 5 minutes at 160 Fahrenheit. Place your fingers in the fry container. Let them cook at the same heat for about fifteen minutes. Toss the fingers well, so they're fried uniformly. Drizzle the garlic paste and serve.

Nutrition: Calories: 160, Fat: 11g, Protein: 12g.

28. Pork Barbecue Sandwich

(Ready in about 1hr 55 min | Servings 4 | Difficult)

Ingredients:

- Two slices of white bread

- 1 tbsp of softened butter

- 1/2 lbs of cut pork (in cubes)

- 1 little capsicum

For sauce barbeque:

- 1/4 tbsp of Worcestershire

- 1/2 tsp of olive oil

- 1/2 crushed garlic flake

- 1/4 cup of onion

- 1/4 tsp of powder mustard

- 1/2 tbsp of sugar

- 1/4 tbsp of hot chili sauce

- 1 tbsp of tomatoes ketchup

- 1/2 cup of water.

- A pinch of salt and black chilies to the taste

Directions:

1. Take the bread slices and cut the rims. Now clean the slices in the horizontal way. Heat the sauce ingredients and wait before sauce thickens.

2. Now fill in the pork into the sauce before it gets its flavors. Stir in the capsicum and Peel off skin. The capsicum is sliced into strips. Combine products. And add it to slices of bread.

3. Preheat the AirFryer to 300 Fahrenheit for 5 minutes. Open the Fryer basket and put the sandwiches prepared in it so that no 2 Sandwiches bump into each other. Now hold the fryer at 250° for Fifteen minutes.

4. Turn the sandwiches in between the cooking to Cook slices of both. Serve the sandwiches with tomato ketchup or chutney.

Nutrition: Calories: 134, Fat: 6g, Protein: 11g.

29. Chili Lamb

(Ready in about 1hr 25 min | Servings 5 | Difficult)

Ingredients:

- 1 lb. of lamb (cut into cubes)

- 2 1/2 tsp of ginger-garlic paste

- 1 tsp of red chili sauce

- 1/4 tsp of salt

- 1/4 tsp of red chili powder / black pepper

- Three drops of orange food coloring

For sauce:

- 2 tbsp of olive oil

- 1 1/2 tsp of ginger garlic paste

- 1/2 tbsp of red chili sauce

- 2 tbsp of tomatoes ketchup

- 2 tsp of soybean sauce

- 1-2 tbsp of honey

- 1/4 tsp of ajinomoto

- 1-2 tsp of red chili flakes

Directions:

1. Combine all the ingredients for marinade and place the cubes of the lamb inside and Let it rest overnight Balance well the flakes of breadcrumbs, oregano, and red chili, and put the marinated fingers on this paste.

2. Cover with plastic wrap and leave before prepared to cook — prefire up the AirFryer for five minutes at 160 Fahrenheit.

3. Place your fingers in and near the fry container. Let them cook at the same heat for fifteen minutes. Toss the fingers well, so they're cooked uniformly.

Nutrition: Calories: 110, Fat: 9g, Protein: 11g.

Chapter 5. Fish and Seafood

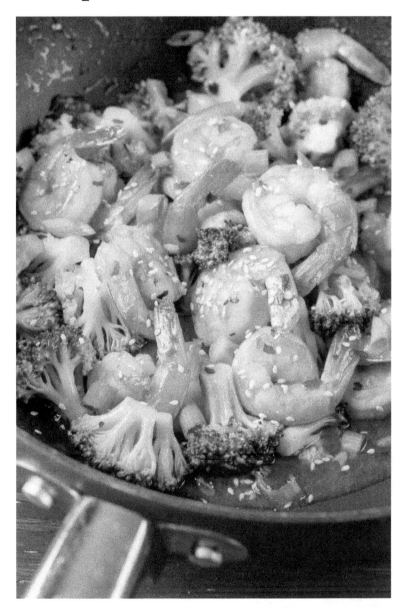

30. Appetizer of Cajun Shrimp

(Ready in about 15 min | Servings 2 | Normal)

Ingredients:

- Twenty tiger shrimps, peeled

- Salt and black chili, to satisfy

- Seasoning with 1/2 teaspoon of old bay

- 1 tablespoon of olive oil

- 1/4 smoked paprika teaspoon

Directions:

1. Comb the shrimps in a bowl with the Fat:, salt, pepper, old bay seasoning, paprika, and toss to coat.

2. Place the shrimp in the basket of your AirFryer and cook at 390 °F for Five minutes.

3. Put them up on a tray and serve as an appetizer.

Enjoy!

Nutrition: Calories: 162, Fat: 6g, Fiber: 4g, Carbohydrates 8g, Protein: 14g.

31. Crispy Shrimps

(Ready in about 15 min | Servings 4 | Normal)

Ingredients:

- 12 large shrimps, dewed and peeled

- 2 white eggs

- 1 cup of crushed coconut

- 1 cup panko crumbs with bread

- 1 coupe of white flour

- Salt and black chili, to try

Directions:

1. Place panko and coconut in a cup, then mix.

2. In a second container, put the rice, salt, and pepper and whisk the egg whites in the third.

3. Sprinkle shrimp in rice, blend egg whites and coconut, put it in your AirFryer pan at 350° F for ten minutes, halfway rolling.

4. Set on a plate and serve as an appetizer.

Enjoy!

Nutrition: Calories: 140, Fat: 4g, Fiber: 0, Carbs: 3g, Protein: 4g.

32. Crab Sticks

(Ready in about 22 min | Servings 4 | Normal)

Ingredients:

- Ten crabsticks, cut by half

- Two sesame seeds teaspoons

- 2 teaspoons of seasoning Cajun

Directions:

1. In a container, place the crab sticks, apply the sesame oil and the Cajun seasoning, toss, transfer

to your AirFryer pan and cook 350° F for 12 Minutes.

2. Organize on a tray and serve as an appetizer.

Enjoy!

Nutrition: Calories: 110, Fat: 0, Fiber: 1g , Carbohydrates 4g, Protein: 2g.

33. Patties in the Salmon Party

(Ready in about 22 min | Servings 4 | Normal)

Ingredients:

- Three big, cooked, drained, and mashed potatoes

- 1 big, skinless, boneless salmon fillet

- 2 tablespoons of parsley, chopped

- 2 tablespoons of dill, chopped

- Salt and black chili, to try

- 1 egg

- 2 spoonsful of bread crumbs

- Cooking spray

Directions:

1. Place salmon in the basket of your AirFryer and cook at 360° F for 10 minutes

2. Transfer the salmon to a baking sheet, cool it, flake it, and drop in a bowl

3. Introduce crumbs of mashed potatoes, salt, pepper, dill, parsley, egg whites, and bread, whisk excellently, and form eight patties out of the mixture.

4. Place salmon patties in the basket of your AirFryer, spray with the cooking oil, cook for 12 minutes at 360 °F, turn them halfway.

5. Serve as an appetizer.

Enjoy!

Nutrition: Calories: 231, Fat: 3g, Fiber: 7g, Carbohydrates 14g, Protein: 4g.

34. Shrimp Muffins

(Ready in about 36 min | Servings 6 | Normal)

Ingredients:

- 1 pound of spaghetti sliced and halved

- 2 tablespoons of mayonnaise

- 1 cup of sliced mozzarella

- Eight shrimp on ounces, peeled, fried, and chopped

- 1 and 1/2 cups of panko

- 1 teaspoon of parsley flakes

- 1 clove of garlic, minced

- Salt and black chili, to try

- Cooking spray

Directions:

1. Place the squash halves in the AirFryer, cook for 16 minutes at 350° F. Set aside to cool off, then brush flesh into a cup.

2. Add salt, chili pepper, parsley flakes, panko, shrimp, and mayo. Stir gently, and add mozzarella.

3. Squirt a muffin tray with a cooking spray that suits your AirFryer and divide each cup into squash and shrimp mixture.

4. Stir in the fryer and cook for 10 minutes at 360° Fahrenheit.

5. Placed muffins on a tray and serve as a snack.

Enjoy it!

Nutrition: Calories: 60, Fat: 2, Carbohydrates 4, Protein: 4, Fiber: 0.4g

Chapter 6. Poultry Recipes

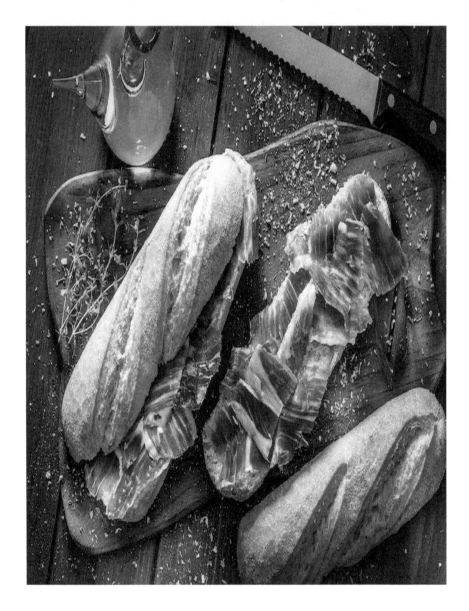

35. Japanese Mixed Chicken

(Ready in about 18 min | Servings 2 | Normal)

Ingredients:

- Two thighs of chicken, skinless and boneless

- Two slices of ginger, chopped

- 3 cloves of garlic, minced

- 1/4 cup of soy sauce

- 1/4 cup of mirin

- 1/8 cup of sake

- 1/2 cubit of sesame oil

- 1/8 cups of water

- 2 spoonfuls of sugar

- 1 spoonful of corn starch mixed with 2 spoonfuls of water

- Sesame seeds to serve

Directions:

1. Mix the chicken thighs in a bowl with the ginger, garlic, soy sauce, mirin, sake, toss well with water, sugar, and cornstarch, switch to preheated AirFryer. Cook for 8 minutes, at 360° F.

2. Sprinkle the sesame seeds on top and serve.

Enjoy it!

Nutrition: Calories: 300, Fat: 7g, Fiber: 9g, Carbs: 17g, Protein: 10g.

36. Succulent Turkey Breast Lunch

(Ready in about 57 min | Servings 4 | Normal)

Ingredients:

- 1 large turkey breast

- 2 tablespoons of olive oil

- 1/2 smoked paprika teaspoon

- 1 tsp of dried thyme

- 1/2 sage teaspoon, dry

- Salt and black chili, to try

- 2 mustard spoons

- 1/4 cup of incredible syrup

- 1 ginger butter, mild

Directions:

1. Rub with the olive oil, season with salt, pepper, thyme. Rub the paprika and sage, put them in the basket of your AirFryer, and fry at 350° F for 25 minutes.

2. Turn turkey, bake for another 10 minutes, turn over again and simmer for maybe another ten minutes.

3. In the meantime, prepare a saucepan over medium heat with butter, add mustard

And the maple syrup, stir well, simmer for a few minutes, and turn off.

4. Break the turkey breast and split it between the bowls.

Enjoy!

Nutrition: Calories: 280, Fat: 2g, fiber 7g, Carbohydrates 16g, Protein: 14g.

37. Cream Chicken Stew

(Ready in about 35 min | Servings 4 | Normal)

Ingredients:

- 1 and 1/2 cups of celery cream

- 6 tenders for chicken

- Salt and black chili, to try

- 2 diced potatoes

- 1 bay leaf

- 1 spring thyme, chopped

- Tsp of milk

- 1 yolk of an egg

- 1/2 cup milk, hard

Directions:

1. Mix the chicken in a bowl of celery cream, rice, oil, bay leaf, thyme, salt, and pepper.S hake, spray in the AirFryer and cook for 25 minutes at 320° F.

2. Let your stew cool off a little, remove the bay leaf, break between pot, and serve promptly.

Enjoy!

Nutrition: Calories: 300, Fat: 11g, Fiber: 2g, Carbohydrates 23g, Protein: 14g.

38. Turkey Cakes

(Ready in about 20 min | Servings 4 | Normal)

Ingredients:

- 6 champignons, split

- 1 teaspoon of crushed garlic

- 1 teaspoon of ground onion

- Salt and black chili, to try

- 1 and 1/4 kg of turkey poultry, ground

- Kitchen spray

- Tomato sauce

Directions:

1. Mix champignons with salt and pepper in your mixer and pulse well, then step into a tub.

2. Whisk and add turkey, onion powder, garlic powder, salt, and pepper made from this blend.

3. Sprinkle with a cooking mist, pass it to the AirFryer and cook for 10 minutes, at 320° F.

4. Serve them side by side with tomato sauce and a savory side salad.

Enjoy!

Nutrition: Calories: 202, Fat: 6g, Fiber: 3g, Carbohydrates 17g, Protein: 10g.

39. Coconut and Casserole Chicken

(Ready in about 35 min | Servings 4 | Normal)

Ingredients:

- Four lime leaves ripped

- 1 cup of vegetable stock

- 1 split stalk of lemongrass,

- 1 pound of chicken breast, skinless, boneless

- 8 ounces of mushrooms

- 4 Thai chilies, sliced

- 4 spoonfuls of fish sauce

- 6 tablespoon of coconut milk

- 1/4 tablespoon of lemon juice

- 1/4 cup of cilantro

- Salt and black chili, to try

Directions:

1. Place stock in a saucepan that blends in with your fryer, push to a boil, add medium fire, lemongrass, lime leaves, ginger, mix and cook for 10 minutes.

2. Strain soup, return to saucepan, add chicken, champignons, rice, chilies, fish, sauce, lime juice, cilantro, salt, chili pepper, stir, place in the fryer. Cook for 15 minutes, at 360° F.

3. Divide in and serve in pots.

Enjoy!

Nutrition: Calories: 150, Fat: 4g, Carbohydrates 4g, Carbohydrates 6g, Protein: 7g.

40. Turkey Burgers

(Ready in about 18 min | Servings 4 | Normal)

Ingredients:

- 1 lb of turquoise beef, ground

- 1 shallot, diced

- A trickle of olive oil

- 1 Thin, chopped jalapeno pepper

- 2 cups of lime juice

- 1 lime zest, grated

- Salt and black chili, to try

- 1 tsp of ground cumin

- 1 tsp of tender paprika

- Guacamole

Directions:

1. Mix the turkey meat in a dish of salt, pepper, cumin, paprika, shallot, jalapeno, lime juice, zest, mix well, type burgers. This blend, spray the oil over them, put in the preheated AirFryer, and cook them on either side for 8 minutes at 370° F.

2. Divide between bowls, then serve on top of the guacamole.

Enjoy!

Nutrition: Calories: 200, Fat: 12g, Fiber: 0, Protein: 12g.

Chapter 7. Desserts and Sweets Recipes

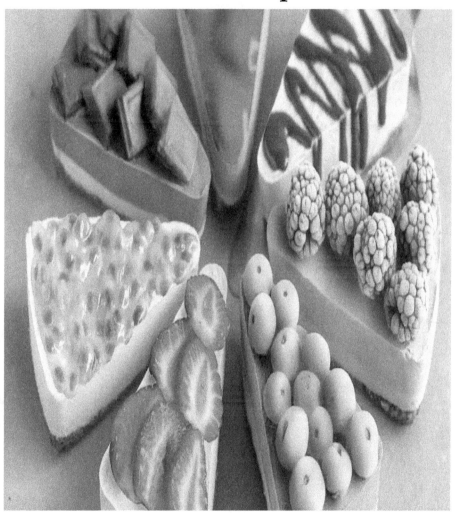

41. Pajamas Jiggery

(Ready in about 15 min | Servings 2 | Normal)

Ingredients:

- 2 cups of milk

- 1 cup of jiggery melted

- 2 tbsp. of custard powder

- 3 tbsp. of glazed sugar

- 3 tbsp. of butter, unsalted

Directions:

1. In a saucepan, boil the milk and the sugar and add the custard powder through the jiggery and whisk until the mixture is thick. You need to stir well.

2. Preheat the Fryer for five minutes to 300 Fahrenheit. Place the platter in the pan basket and cool down to 250 Fahrenheit cook for ten mines and left alone to get cool down.

Nutrition: Calories: 5, Fat: 6g, Protein: 11g.

42. Semolina Pudding

(Ready in about 15 min | Servings 2 | Normal)

Ingredients:

- 2 cups of milk

- 2 tbsp. of custard powder

- Three tbsp. of glazed sugar

- 2 tbsp. of semolina

- 3 tbsp. of butter, unsalted

Directions:

1. In a saucepan, boil the milk and sugar, add the custard powder and mix until prepared. Apply the semolina to the saucepan and ensure the mixture is becoming somewhat thicker.

2. Preheat the Fryer for five minutes to 300 Fahrenheit. Place the platter in the pan basket and cool down to 250 Fahrenheit. Heat 10 minutes and let it cool down.

Nutrition: Calories: 34, Fat: 9g, Protein: 13g.

43. Date Waffles

(Ready in about 18 min | Servings 8 | Normal)

Ingredients:

- 3 cups of almond meal

- 3 eggs

- 2 tsp. of dry basil

- 2 tsp. of dried parsley

- Salt and pepper

- 3 tbsp. of butter

- 2 cups of dates, pitted and diced

Directions:

1. The AirFryer is preheated to 250 Fahrenheit. Mix the ingredients, except the dates, in a shallow dish. Check it's a smooth and well-balanced blend.

2. Take a buttered waffle mold, then grate it. Apply the mound to the batter and put it in the basket of an AirFryer. Cook until all sides tan. Try to create a cavity, and fill with dates.

Nutrition: Calories: 232, Fat: 4g, Protein: 4g.

44. Pudding Times

(Ready in about 15 min | Servings 2 | Normal)

Ingredients:

- 2 tbsp. of powder custard

- 3 tbsp. of glazed sugar

- 3 tbsp. of butter unsalted

- 1 cup of dates pitted and diced

Directions:

1. In a saucepan, boil the milk and the sugar and incorporate the custard powder rile up by the dates before you have a thick blend. Pour in the sliced fruits and Blend.

2. Preheat the Fryer for five minutes to 300 Fahrenheit. Place the platter in the pan basket and cool down to 250 Fahrenheit. Heat 10 minutes and set to cool down.

Nutrition: Calories: 60, Fat: 12g, Protein: 3g.

45. Mediterranean Splendor

(Ready in about 18 min | Servings 5 | Normal)

Ingredients:

- 2 cups of milk

- 2 cups of almond flour

- 2 tbsp. of mine custard

- 3 tbsp. of glazed sugar

- 3 tbsp. of butter unsalted

- 2 cups of mix Mediterranean fruit

Directions:

1. In a saucepan, heat the milk and the sugar and incorporate the custard powder. Comb with the almond flour and mix until the paste is thick. Add in the fruit mixture in the bowl.

2. Preheat the Fryer for five minutes to 300 Fahrenheit. Place the platter in the pan basket and cool down to 250 Fahrenheit. Heat 10 minutes and ready to cool down.

Nutrition: Calories: 98, Fat: 42g, Protein: 33g.

46. Pudding of Guava

(Ready in about 12 min | Servings 3 | Normal)

Ingredients:

- 2 cups of butter

- 2 cups of almond flour

- Two tbsp. of mine custard

- Three tbsp. of glazed sugar

- Three tbsp. of butter unsalted

- 2 cups of pulp guava

Directions:

1. In a saucepan, heat the milk and the sugar and incorporate the custard powder. Comb with the almond flour and whisk until the paste is thick. Mix in the guava pulp to the combination.

2. Preheat the Fryer for five minutes to 300 Fahrenheit. Place the platter in the pan basket and

cool down to 250 Fahrenheit. Heat 10 minutes and ready to cool down.

Nutrition: Calories: 50, Fat: 34g, Protein: 12g.

47. Passion Fruit Pudding

(Ready in about 20 min | Servings 4 | Normal)

Ingredients:

- 2 cups of almond flour

- 2 cups of milk

- 2 cups of passion fruit pulp

- 2 tbsp. of mine custard

- 3 tbsp. of glazed sugar

- 3 tbsp. of butter, unsalted

Directions:

1. In a saucepan, simmer the milk and the sugar and incorporate the custard powder and flour and whisk until the mixture is thick. Finely chop the apricot and Throw into the mix.

2. Preheat the Fryer for five minutes to 300 Fahrenheit. Place the platter in the pan basket and

cool down to 250 Fahrenheit. Heat 10 minutes and ready to cool down. Cover the fruit over the bread and serve.

Nutrition: Calories: 50, Fat: 24g, Protein: 2g.

48. Blackcurrant Pudding

(Ready in about 20 min | Servings 4 | Normal)

Ingredients:

- 2 cups of milk

- 2 cups of almond flour

- 2 tbsp. of mine custard

- 3 tbsp. of glazed sugar

- 1 cup of pulp with black currant

- 3 tbsp. of butter unsalted

Directions:

1. In a saucepan, simmer the milk and the sugar and incorporate the custard powder. Comb with the almond flour and stir until the paste is thick. Slice the figs fine and then apply it to the blend.

2. Preheat the Fryer for five minutes to 300 Fahrenheit. Place the platter in the pan basket and

cool down to 250 Fahrenheit. Heat 10 minutes and set to cool down.

Nutrition: Calories: 43, Fat: 23g, Protein: 12g.

Chapter 8. Lunch Recipes

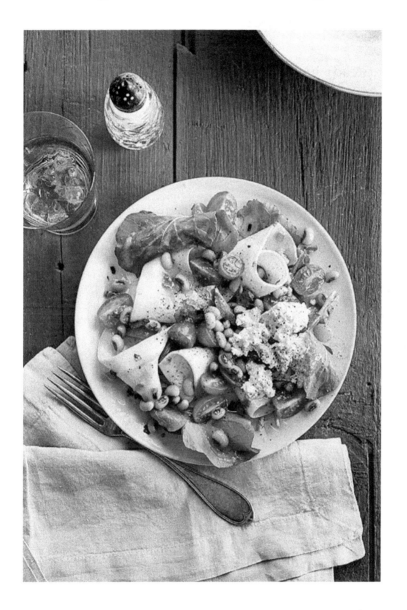

49. Whole-Wheat Pizzas in an AirFryer

(Ready in about 35 min | Servings 2 | Normal)

Ingredients:

- ¼ cup of lower-Sodium marinara sauce

- 2 whole-wheat pita rounds

- 1 cup of baby spinach leaves (1 oz.)

- 1 small plum tomato, cut into 8 slices

- 1 small garlic clove, thinly sliced

- 1-ounce of pre-shredded part-skim mozzarella cheese (about 1/4 cup)

- ¼ ounce of shaved Parmigiano-Reggiano cheese (about 1 Tbsp.)

Directions:

1. Layer the marinara sauce uniformly over 1 side of each pita. Cover the spinach leaves with quarters, tomato slices, garlic, and cheeses.

2. Put 1 pita in an AirFryer basket and cook at 350° F for 4 to 5 minutes until cheese is melted and pita is crisp. Repeat with pita left over.

Nutrition: Calories: 229, Fat: 5g, Protein: 11g, Carbohydrate: 37g, Fiber: 5g, Sugars: 4g, Added Sugars: 0g, Sodium: 510mg, Calcium: 18%.

50. Prosciutto Sandwich

(Ready in about 15 min | Servings 1 | Normal)

Ingredients:

- 2 bread slices

- 2 mozzarella slices

- 2 tomato slices

- 2 prosciutto slices

- 2 basil leaves

- 1 teaspoon of olive oil

- A pinch of salt and black pepper

Directions:

1. Arrange mozzarella and prosciutto on a bread slice.

2. Season with salt and pepper, place in your AirFryer and cook at 400° F for 5 minutes.

3. Drizzle oil over prosciutto, add tomato and basil, cover with the other bread slice, cut the sandwich in half and serve.

Enjoy!

Nutrition: Calories: 172, Fat: 3g, Fiber: 7g, Carbs: 9g, Protein: 5g.

Conclusion

Anything you can imagine, from chicken to French fries to fish, can be made healthier in an air fryer because its cooking method requires very little fat. For example, a batch of French fries requires only half a tablespoon of oil and 12 minutes to serve crisp. Similarly, an air fryer prepares burgers, steaks, and fries in just a few minutes. You'll be surprised, but in just 25 minutes, you can bake an entire pie in an air fryer!

The exhaust system controls the temperature, which is increased by internal pressure and emits additional air as needed to cook the food. The extra air is completely filtered before being released, making it better for the environment. Air fryers are both environmentally and user friendly.

CPSIA information can be obtained
at www.ICGtesting.com
Printed in the USA
BVHW062336010321
601388BV00009B/985